A Possible Trust
The Poetry of Ronna Bloom

T0355817

A Possible Trust
The Poetry of Ronna Bloom

Selected
with an
introduction by
Phil Hall
and an
afterword by
Ronna Bloom

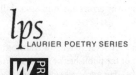
lps
LAURIER POETRY SERIES

WLU PRESS
WILFRID LAURIER
UNIVERSITY PRESS

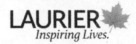

Wilfrid Laurier University Press acknowledges the support of the Canada Council for the Arts for our publishing program. We acknowledge the financial support of the Government of Canada through the Canada Book Fund for our publishing activities. Funding provided by the Government of Ontario and the Ontario Arts Council. This work was supported by the Research Support Fund.

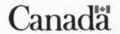 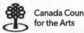

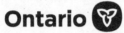 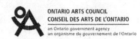

Library and Archives Canada Cataloguing in Publication

Title: A possible trust : the poetry of Ronna Bloom / selected with an introduction by Phil Hall and an afterword by Ronna Bloom.
Other titles: Poems. Selections
Names: Bloom, Ronna, 1961– author. | Hall, Phil, 1953– editor. | Bloom, Ronna, writer of afterword.
Series: Laurier poetry series.
Description: Series statement: Laurier poetry series | Includes bibliographical references.
Identifiers: Canadiana (print) 20220498210 | Canadiana (ebook) 20220498253 | ISBN 9781771125956 (softcover) | ISBN 9781771125963 (EPUB) | ISBN 9781771125970 (PDF)
Classification: LCC PS8553.L665 A6 2023 | DDC C811/.54—dc23

Front cover image: *Blue Grit* by Tim Deverell.
Cover design by Gary Blakeley.
Interior design by Mike Bechthold.

© 2023 Wilfrid Laurier University Press
Waterloo, Ontario, Canada
www.wlupress.wlu.ca

This book is printed on FSC®certified paper, contains post-consumer fiber and other controlled sources, is manufactured using renewable energy-biogas and processed chlorine free.

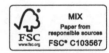

Printed in Canada

Wilfrid Laurier University Press is located on the Haldimand Tract, part of the traditional territories of the Haudenosaunee, Anishnaabe, and Neutral Peoples. This land is part of the Dish with One Spoon Treaty between the Haudenosaunee and Anishnaabe Peoples and symbolizes the agreement to share, to protect our resources, and not to engage in conflict. We are grateful to the Indigenous Peoples who continue to care for and remain interconnected with this land. Through the work we publish in partnership with our authors, we seek to honour our local and larger community relationships, and to engage with the diversity of collective knowledge integral to responsible scholarly and cultural exchange.

Table of Contents

Foreword, *Tanis MacDonald* / ix
Biographical Note / xi
Introduction: "To Lead by Crying," *Phil Hall* / xv

from *Fear of the Ride*
The City / 3
Here / 4
The Job on an Apple / 5

from *Personal Effects*
Truth and Reconciliation / 6
Personal Effects / 7
Just This / 11

from *Public Works*
What Works / 12
Work / 14
Goodbye to All the Rooms / 15
Everybody's Birds / 16
A Possible Trust / 18

from *Permiso*
Water / 20
Permiso / 21
The Leash / 22

from *Cloudy with a Fire in the Basement*
The Parade / 23
The Peace You Are Waiting For / 24
Grief Without Fantasy / 25
Preserves / 26
Use These Poems / 27
The Spontaneous Poetry Booth / 28

from *The Spontaneous Poetry Booth*
Molecular / 29
Don't Be Superficial, 'Cause We'll Soon Find Out / 30

from *The More*
Ars Poetica / 31
Why Are You So Scared? / 32
Appointment in Samarra / 33
Ethel / 34
Rest / 35
Health / 36
Walking the Hospital / 40
The More / 43

from *Who is your mercy contact?*
Bukowski / 44
Service / 45
Immeasurable / 46

New Work
Clothes / 47

Afterword, "To Connect Is a Circular Thing," Ronna Bloom / 49
Notes and Acknowledgements / 55

Foreword

I am happy to serve as the general editor for the Laurier Poetry Series, the development and growth of which I have followed from its early days. My gratitude goes to Neil Besner and Brian Henderson, who conceived of the Laurier Poetry Series in 2002 as a way to offer a more robust selection of a single poet's work than could be found in an anthology. In 2004, the Laurier Poetry Series launched the first volume, Catherine Hunter's selection of the poems of Lorna Crozier, *Before the First Word*. Neil served as General Editor for all volumes until he was joined in 2016 by Brian, when he left his role as WLU Press's Director. In an act of commitment to poetry publication that is nothing short of inspiring, the Laurier Poetry Series expanded to a list of thirty-three fascinating titles under their leadership.

The retirement of the original editors has given me a surprising historical jolt. But thinking historically is a good way to revisit the original plans for the series, and to think towards the future. Under my editorial eye, the series will retain its original aim to produce volumes of poetry made widely available to new readers, including undergraduate students at universities or colleges, and to a general readership who wish for "more poetry in their poetry." WLU Press also retains its commitment to produce beautiful volumes and to alert readers to poems that remain vital to thinking about urgencies of the contemporary moment. It is a reality that poetry books are produced in smaller print runs and often on a shoestring, and as a consequence, original collections of poetry tend to go out of print too quickly and far too precipitously. The series has the added goal of bringing poems from out-of-print collections back into the public eye and the public discourse. The Press's commitment to the work of literary studies includes choosing editors for each volume who can reflect deeply on the body of work, as well as inviting original afterwords from the poets themselves.

As we embark on this next turn of the series, access is our watchword. Canadian literature has undeniably had a checkered history of exclusionary practices, so who gets the nod and who takes part in discussions—as readers and as writers—of Canadian poetry? In the classroom, it is my privilege and my task to introduce a generation of students to the practice of reading poetry as a vital thread in cultural, social, and political conversations, conversations that challenge ideas about Canada and seek to illuminate and bring to consciousness better futures. For that work, I want access to as many voices on the page, and as robust a selection of poems from those voices, as I can get my hands on. This is the language of the bibliophile, the craver of books, the person whose pedagogical pleasure comes from putting poetry books into the hands of others and saying, simply, "Read this, and we'll talk." Multi-author anthologies do not always usefully demonstrate to readers how a poet's work shifts and changes over the years, nor do they always display the ways that a single poet's poems speak to and with and sometimes usefully against one another. I want at my elbow, in every discussion, inside and outside the classroom, our best poetic practitioners. I want books that offer not just a few poems, but dozens: selected volumes not only by the splashiest prize winners but also significantly by poets who have been carrying a full cultural backpack for decades. I also want to showcase new and prolific voices who have taken off like rockets. For this, I am grateful for the chance to bring these poets to you, or bring them back to you. Turn is sometimes a return and sometimes a revolution. Neil and Brian started this series off with a bang, and now it's time to light another fuse.

The volume you hold in your hands sizzles. Read this, and we'll talk.

—*Tanis MacDonald*
General Editor

Biographical Note

Ronna Bloom was born in Montreal, went to Hebrew Day School, and received a BA in Film and Philosophy from Clark University in Worcester, Massachusetts.

For three years in the 1980s, she lived in the West of Ireland as a photographer, working with Ron Rosenstock in the Irish Photographic Workshop and exhibiting her photographs and photo-text pieces in Westport, Galway, and Dublin.

Later, she spent two years in London, England where she received a Higher Diploma in Fine Art from the Slade School of Art. She made performance videos in which she sat in front of a camera and told stories, somewhat in the manner of Spalding Gray. Her video, "I feel hopeful about the future," toured widely in Europe and is distributed by Cinenova and LUX, and is housed at the British Film Institute National Archive.

She received her MEd in Counselling Psychology at the Ontario Institute for Studies in Education, and worked as a psychotherapist for 25 years. For twelve years she worked in Counselling and Learning Skills Services at University of Toronto.

In 1980, she worked as a volunteer at the American Film Institute on a celebration of women in film—and met Lillian Gish. In 1986, she attended a reading by Audre Lorde, who pierced the unconscious bubble in which she lived by saying to the audience, "know where your power is." Around 2000, she heard Clifton Joseph perform "Chant for Monk" at the Scream in High Park and he blew the park open. These three moments were liberating for her.

Between 1996 and 2017, she published six books of poems, five with Pedlar Press and one with Carleton University Press, now in the hands of McGill-Queen's University Press. Discovering her better methods from book to book, she has struggled between scouring poems for truth—or being nice, writing poems that are friendly, funny—and has chosen to make luminous poems that accommodate both truth and generosity.

She has been comforted, awoken, melted, infused, and rocked by the work of her literary aunts, uncles, cousins: Adrienne Rich, Lucille Clifton, Jim Harrison, Rumi, Hafiz, Laurie Anderson, Raymond Carver, Rainer Maria Rilke, Yoko Ono. In Canada, she has been inspired by Rhea Tregebov, Erín Moure, Roo Borson, and Maureen Hynes.

In 2008, Ronna developed the Poet and Community Program at the University of Toronto. She offered workshops through which students explored their personal, academic, social, and spiritual selves through poetry. This program ran until 2022.

In 2010, Ronna began to practice meditation in the Dzogchen tradition of Tibetan Buddhism.

In 2012, she created the Poet in Residence Program at Sinai Health in Toronto, leading writing workshops for staff, patients, and visitors. Part of her offerings included The Spontaneous Poetry Booth, where she would write a poem on the spot for any person in need.

"What do you need a poem for?" she would ask people who lined up at her booth. Then she would sit with each person quietly, and talk awhile, until the first line came. She would write their poem, read it out loud, and then hand it to them. At another version of the booth, called *Rx for Poetry*, Ronna would prescribe poems (printed on prescription pads) by Langston Hughes, Emily Dickinson, Hafiz, and others.

She has given talks on poetry in health care and offered The Spontaneous Poetry Booth and the Rx for Poetry booth at universities, hospitals, conferences, and fundraisers in Canada, Italy, and the UK (including PEN Canada and Freedom from Torture).

Ronna has collaborated with architects, filmmakers, academics, musicians, choreographers, conservationists, and spiritual leaders. In 2018, her poem "The City" was painted on King Street in Toronto in a public art project by PLANT Architects.

Her books have been shortlisted for the Gerald Lampert Award, the Pat Lowther Award, and the ReLit Award, and longlisted for the City of Toronto Book Award. Her poetry has been recorded for the Canadian National Institute for the Blind, and translated into Spanish, Chinese, and Bangla. Ronna's chapbook, *Who is your mercy contact?*, was published by Espresso Chapbooks in 2022.

Bibliography

Fear of the Ride (McGill-Queen's University Press, 1996)
Personal Effects (Pedlar Press, 2000)
Public Works (Pedlar Press, 2004)
Permiso (Pedlar Press, 2009)
Cloudy with a Fire in the Basement (Pedlar Press, 2012)
The More (Pedlar Press, 2017)
Who is your mercy contact? (Espresso, 2022)

Introduction

To Lead by Crying

Ronna Bloom makes useful poems that while struggling with hope are able to offer hope.

"Look at this photograph," says Ronna.

In the photo she hands me, a woman in a hospital corridor has just received a spontaneous poem from Bloom—and the look on the woman's face is so grateful, so opened out and away from trouble, for a moment at least.

Or her trouble is with her still, but she is carrying it better now, after receiving the poem, and she is beautiful in her fortitude and gratitude.

When poetry strives to be a healing art, it favours no personae—except the personae of the letters themselves.

Each letter (even when cursive) is a mask that a natural process wears in order to reach us, and reach through us—so perhaps we need no other disguises.

No personae, then, and no pride in form or mystery. No system. No obscurantics. Ronna Bloom's poems offer an art with no evasion, no exo-system, no aloofness.

She offers a *nowness*. Which can be scary—how next will we be called upon by this poet, line by line?

She increasingly writes poems in which mystery has its foundations in a collective self, and in the poet's complicated connection to that collective self.

The lab coat worn by the poet in the hospital would suggest a persona, but can an art of honesty sustain a persona?

The Rx Poetry Pad—*here's your prescription, here's your poem*—well, all that's a bit of a gimmick, sure—a prop to go with the costume.

Or are these props actually vehicles of risk? A way to make light of raw risk. Toward making daily light. On the patient's part and on the poet's part. An exchange of risk. In hope of a possible trust.

Here's one of the Poetry Booth poems: "Fear." In its natural state, it is in cursive...

> When I strip away
> all I thought that made me
> something, and take off the garments
> of history,
> I stand almost naked
> at the crossroads
> heartshaking open
> getting ready
> getting free.

One sentence. One stanza. Simple words. Standard metaphors. Repetition. Old tools. A gift given.

But there are three deepening moments here. We may almost miss them as they deepen us.

When "made me" changes to "made me / something" by enjambment we exit the ego.

When the word "history" enters the poem, it widens.

When "getting ready" doesn't specify what is being gotten ready for, by that discretion we overextend—into that anticipation which is lyric poise.

Why has Ronna Bloom been drawn to hospitals? No one can easily imagine a poet-in-residence in a lawyer's office.

Why? Because poetry is not naturally drawn to deliberation, it is drawn to suffering, to crisis and disaster, to pain.

Why? Because the quick of experience abides at the inexpressible. And right there, at the inexpressible, is language's challenge.

Bloom has been pulled into service at the site of the inexpressible. Not into sentimentality, nor popular tenderness, nor pity.

It is not clean, easy, or fancy to dwell on all this anguish. But a poetry that is willing to know pain, loss, and death may be able to give, if not cessation, at least company—by words.

Bloom wants to be a passing cause of our happiness too. Her voice wants to be the voice of The Friend that Hafiz refers to, and also at times The Sin-Eater, who says, "I've had to swallow that too."

And she wants to be funny in our company, as if giving Empathy bubbles. She can be the clown of her own poem.

And these are urban poems. Ronna Bloom *is* "The City." She is Yonge Street as she drives up it.

She looks down the length of herself and sees her toes as off-ramps onto interchanges speeding away. There is a *teemingness* in her poems.

And an isolation. These are lyrics, after all, and this is what lyrics do. Many of her poems come from solo moments, are creature cries.

Not a phone call, but a small song spinning in its juices, asking for nothing. For everything. When Bloom says "to survive is not to answer," this is both advice, and a note to self.

Bloom has been the watcher at the translator's party, or at the writer's colony, but she has also been up too late and needing the woman across the way to be up and at her window too.

"Beethoven, Rilke, Rumi, Hafiz . . . and no one no one no one no one."

Also notice that these poems are not repositories of information. They do not lead with research about hot or obscure topics. They rarely use medical jargon. They have no embellished diagnoses.

Even the prose poem "Walking the Hospital"—after wading into hospital troubles such as "chemo, ortho, maxillofacial"—ends at another lay question, another desperate prayer:

"If each one poem, person, experience, identity, thought, bone, body—like a point of light—is just itself, does it need a story to connect it to the next one? Awareness, carry me."

Surely it is a patient talking here, not an authority. Whereby does light come from among us—and how can it be shared immediately, without preamble, or cant?

Once Bloom was asked (oddly) before a workshop, "What is your leadership model?" Her reply was, "I lead by crying!"

Or she will say in a poem, "I am a big crier. / And angry." Notice the anger, it inflames and purifies tears. It puts the torch to words to temper them.

These are an angry woman's poems. Or they sing a reconciled woman's blues. These poems speak to us all, but maybe to women first.

The old women of culture come back, feed us, tell us where we came from.

And Bloom speaks to those who are right in front of her, then only later does she speak to us readers of her books.

This woman is not walking away. Down the hallways we are parked in she comes, dragging common language to us—by its jubilant snout.

Why is she asking us so many questions all the time? Because she is inviting us into the dialectic and the gab-fest.

Bloom has a way of presenting arbitrariness as a fully planned gift. *Did she just write this down (for me alone) impromptu?*

Yes, it seems she did—the poem acts like an easy-going but feisty and full commitment to us in our need.

Or—when she isn't in her Spontaneous Poetry Booth—has Bloom tooled the living heck into these poems to get them just right? Yes, it seems so, also.

We have all come out of the same workshops in which improvement is the *modus*, not improvisation—so the truly spontaneous is rare.

A few poets—Ronna Bloom is one—give us songs that have a tone of impromptu closeness, whether they are tooled or not. They are usually a bit of both.

Bloom gives us a spontaneity that is shared. By being unguarded, by being an unguarded reader, did I just help her write this poem for me? Yep.

In Bloom's case, *craft* is almost—dare I say it—love.

She wants us *not* to observe her skill, but to participate in her discoveries. She wants us *with* her, not appraising her—*love*.

Earlier, I mentioned Bloom's desire to be useful. This is important. Useful, as in keeping separate and thereby having something to give.

But there is here also a desire to be merely one of the tired workers who can still crack a dumb joke to lighten the mood.

As you can tell by now, I too love Ronna Bloom's poems—because there is a *cringe* that becomes a *hinge* in many of them—she will include in a poem her own impatience with herself or her language.

She will cringe from what she tells us, and this will become the poem's hinge into its revelations.

In this book's title, and in the title poem "A Possible Trust," the important word is not "trust" but that qualifying yet optimistic word "possible."

"If thou has fear / thou has company." That is Martin Buber's "thou." How simply said, and how difficult to say. But Bloom says it.

Notice, though, that the verb is not "hath" to match that "thou." The verb is our plainer "has." So harking back, or harking upward, happens right here.

When she works in sequence, the poems are neighbourhood surveys, a series of portraits, public works reports, personal interviews or inventories.

Bloom has published six books of poems, and an arc can be seen from her first, *Fear of the Ride*, to her latest, *The More*.

If we only focus on covers, we see an amusement park ride for the first book—and the illuminated light and radiance of a Rothko painting, all bright yellow, for the latest.

From fear to light—the crest of the arc, the turn in the *raison* of the Poem, the emergence of a distinctive Bloom poem—happens in *Permiso* and then increasingly in *Cloudy with a Fire in the Basement*.

There is a widening, a loosening, a greater sureness. The poems stop aiming to please, and thereby give us more.

What have we mostly left out of this selection: early poems about family, origins, travel; occasional poems; my-lover-left-me poems; I-don't-spend-much-time-in-the-country poems.

My mother's chairs. The house misses you. A Jewish woman resents Christmas. "Israel in the Movies."

As with origins, sexuality is also always nearby, whether mentioned in a poem or not. The rude body. Need. Impatience.

We have to get over ourselves somehow—this is implied. I hate what happened—this is said.

Defiant, comical, revealing, impolite yet respectful poems.

We have left out tributary poems. Instead, we have chosen poems that show the breakthroughs, the trajectory, and the hesitant rush beyond all that.

In choosing poems, we used one innovation—at the poet's suggestion, we put out an invitation to Ronna's colleagues—doctors, nurses, patients, social workers—and to Ronna's friends and poet friends: "Which poems by this poet have been most important to you?"

There was a strong response. We included the poems that got the most endorsements. This collaborative method has seemed in keeping with the intent and import of Bloom's poems. And it speaks to community.

We have also included a couple examples of poems written from the Spontaneous Poetry Booth. We get to see Bloom (in her white lab coat with her Rx Poetry Pad) in her booth at the hospital.

When you hear that the poet has worked as a therapist, don't be fooled into thinking that this full voice is for guidance. Take the good lines away with you, but don't forget their context.

Out of respect for us, and out of respect for the Poem too—Bloom speaks neither from the couch nor the big chair. Part of her gift to us is to be just here with us. With herself too. No furniture. Ready.

Also, don't make the mistake of thinking that a Ronna Bloom poem is necessarily a safe space, as if it involved no challenge.

On YouTube, and at her website, we can watch Bloom toss a whole manuscript into the air (link in Notes and Acknowledgements, at back of book).

She is willing to read the pattern of how it all falls as evidence. She is willing to trust how things fall. Or is she?

If you are looking for Mary Oliver, you will find someone less polite, less formal. Maybe Sappho was this kind of woman. Sharon Olds would be closer. C. D. Wright would be closer.

Bloom is also a populist: "Work" and "How it Works" and "Public Works"—so we might hear the spirit of Dorothy Livesay—a documentary style in defense of "anyone willing."

"Just This" and "Here" and "Truth and Reconciliation"—but don't kid yourself that language is only being used as a method of transfer. Bloom knows that "even the word leashless has a leash in it."

And a word like her fine word "uncovenanted" does not come cheap, ever.

We are told to use these poems "across the sentient grid." As in: stay awake, here it all comes.

If we look at a recent poem, "Service," and consider how it works, we can better know the language care involved:

> The doctors are writing poetry.
> The poets are listening to the stories of soldiers.
> The soldiers are changing the sheets of the aged.
> The aged are dying as trumpetlessly as ever.
>
> And if you could rub their feet,
> that may be all you can do, but it is a lot.
> Their feet get very cold where they are going
> and then get very still.

The end-stop lines are what we notice first. It is an orator's method. Robert Bly uses it to effect in most of his poems.

In this poem we have end stops throughout the first stanza, then one comma in the second. And the final two lines are an open line break moving easily to the last line.

Notice how each line, though, is woven into the next line, so that "poetry" in the first line leads to "poets" in the second, and "soldiers" in the second line leads to soldiers "changing" in the third line.

The soldiers are changing by "changing the sheets of the aged." Everyone in the first stanza is doing something uncharacteristic of their calling.

Even the aged are dying "trumpetlessly." That word is one of the surprises of the poem. It is not what we expected.

We do associate dying soldiers with trumpets, though Bloom says they never have gotten their full honours that way.

Maybe to be listened to, and to have their feet rubbed, is enough. A higher honour.

The poet, though, does not say this is "a higher honour." She says—flatly, unartistically—it is "a lot." And that "a lot" is sopping!

The second last line is the clincher: "Their feet get very cold where they are going." Again, we are not told where the feet will be going. Discretion.

But there is another line, a last line. It is almost too much, it is too much, we know where the feet are going—don't take us there.

But Bloom overdoes it, she takes us there. The poem has to end, the elderly die, soldiers caring for the elderly die—"and then get very still." It is inevitable, that line. It has to be there, whether we like it or not.

A poem like this makes criticism irrelevant, for it is too close to folk wisdom. Its music comes out of interconnections that are not calculating, and that are dormant until sung.

In her most recent poems, we are invited to watch the poet's process as she explores and changes direction—the poem surprising itself in front of us.

There comes a further recognition of the chorus or choir we are all members of. The solo further acknowledges and honours the ensemble.

On Ronna Bloom Street there are wider boulevards—and solidarity. The poems—always very personal—are becoming wider than the personal.

As she says when taking on the personality-driven poetry of Bukowski— "Everybody knows they're nobody. / Why is that such a problem for us?"

From deep isolation in that "nobody," an inclusive "we" is Bloom's subject. Each poem's movement is from "I" to "we."

Her readers are her language, her workshop, her mentors, and her collaborators.

"The conversation / with silence tapped out / like an invisible ink, held to light."

—*Phil Hall*

A Possible Trust

The City

A network of roads spreads finely
through fields, between tower blocks
and building sites, it spins
through highways and downtowns
and downtowns. Dangerous neighbourhoods
await arteries. Maps
the city Toronto to the city Dublin to the city London.
All converge.
Circle road, Ring road.

I am going out all the exits on the highway
at the same time. Mapping
a leg to a shoulder, a memory to a hill, a blue vein
to an arm. Cross
sections of past. Yonge Street meets
King north of Piccadilly Circus
like a skin graft. Major intersections
cross the body.

I don't know where I'm going and the city
calls to my voices, my limbs,
all my uncertain directions, saying:
Lie down in the not knowing.
Lie down in me.

Here

My friend Joe's been dead twelve years
he's used to it already.

Me, I'm scared to meet him after all this time.
"A-1 number 57. Turn left at the oak."

Behind my lids his picture
fixes and unfixes itself

and I tell him, I miss his softness.
You can have it,

he says. Here.

The Job of an Apple

The job of an apple is to be hard,
to be soft, to be crisp, to be red,
yellow and green. The job of an apple is to be pie,
to be given to the teacher, to be rotten.
The job of an apple is to be bad
and good, to be peeled, cored, cut,
bitten and bruised. The job
of an apple is to pose for painters,
roll behind fridges, behind grocery aisles,
to be hidden, wrapped in paper,
stored for months, brought out in the dry heat
of India and eaten like a treasure.
The job of an apple is to be
handed over in orchards, to be wanted
and forbidden. The job of an apple is to be Golden
Delicious, Granny Smith and crab. The job
of an apple is to be imported, banned and confiscated
going through customs from Montreal to New York.
The job of an apple is to be round. Grow. Drop.
To go black in the middle when cut. To be thrown
at politicians. To be carried around for days. To change
hands, to change hands, to change hands.
The job of an apple is to be a different poem in the mouth
of every eater. The job of an apple is to be juice.

Truth and Reconciliation

Our country chose a middle way
of individual amnesty for truth.
                    —Archbishop Desmond Tutu

This man knows something
about healing. That the heart
must be torn open again
in front of compassionate witnesses.
That the accused must also step up
and reveal themself.
That no matter how high-pitched
the shrieks, how barren
the voice, everything must be
heard, everything must be
held, in the same room.

Personal Effects

There are other people's memories in street lights
at the corner of Yonge and Dundas or under the
expressway. Other people's memories are flicked on
passing hospitals and alleyways.
In Vancouver, the voices of teenage girls
are broadcast in the street, telling of boyfriends
and what they wanted or didn't want to do,
whispered over loudspeakers at construction sites.
A certain colour car, a certain make;
this type of pen was a weapon once,
the smell of donuts only a prelude.

Other people's memories go down hot like a swallow
forced in the mouth. Another gag another
woman remembers everything.
She sits with the policeman, the crown
attorney and the friend. The crown says
tell me what you remember, and she can
recount the time on the clock as she sat in the October
car, the colour of upholstery (brown), her foot on the dash,
the man beside and the hand that came from
the back seat, its fingers holding a pen like a knife.
She has a memory for details
and the crown, also a woman, asks
why she removed her dress herself,
why would she do that?
And her memories leave
in the bodies of the police, the crown,
the friend, and herself, as they walk out the door
and go the four winds, each with their own
version, their own retelling or silence.

On Bloor Street near Holt Renfrew
there's a woman begging in a wheelchair.
Stroke melted the brain and the body followed.
Blue sweatpants, palm out. She remembers
nothing. But a woman she meets there
remembers her, remembers her for her,
remembers her once in a spring dress, springy

but she doesn't remember her back. Mouths
words and palms the change.
Now the woman walking away carries
the other's memories, like personal effects
and the wheelchair goes off, glad
of a few dollars to buy lamb chops for dinner.

Other people's memories are passed
by mouth to ear, they enter seamless
and smooth as a ripple of water,
laying itself down like a layer of earth, strata
of the mind, the rings of a tree, or the crusted
bog with its rich sediment below ready
to be cut and dried and burnt.
Another layer of memory is outside
the pool hall and another around the edge
of the pool. *It was a hot day, everyone
was going topless, everyone. Or, it was a summer
night, we all got drunk and went in.
It was there at the park with the shirt
that doesn't button well, he barely
touched it, all the buttons came undone,
the jean jacket I never took off again.
They were my friends I thought
and then they were gone, or else they
were making out under the trees.*
The smell of barbecue chips and silver foil
in the sun.

Other people's memories wait in line
at the Scott Mission, on good days
they are dishing up the meat.

There are memories
on the street that curves called Spadina Crescent,
a cardboard box bends around blankets
to make a paper cave that blows away
in the January snow. The man there, gone too,
afraid of dinners, says someone put a computer chip
in his brain, he was waiting in the boxes, *please come
and get it out.*

The world, he says. *No, no, not the world.*

The ink of the mind is coming through the watering can
brain, making those fantastic Spirograph spirals
of colour, the orange and the blue. He is leaking.
Like watching film on fire: the whole picture dissolving
from the centre. How the film gets stuck
in the projector, the bulb gets too hot
and it doesn't move. It doesn't move
it doesn't move.

What else is there to do but guess,
a history: a piece of clothing in a bag, a neatly folded
shirt, a green baseball cap, a father,
a mother once, they were singers
or bankers, they owned a store on Barton,
they lived in the suburbs
of Montreal, they lived in Victoria.
It was hereditary, it was genetic,
it was the frozen hose against the side of the head,
it was two fingers
between the legs,
they had a house on a hill overlooking the waterworks.
There are memories in the waterworks, under
the marble floor. They are embedded there,
or flow out into the lake or
get turned into novels you can never forget.
People will tell you if you listen.
If they can.
Then every time you pass there, every single time,
you'll be haunted by something
that never happened
to you. But hearing it becomes yours,
seeps into your insides marbling you
so that Yonge Street is a landmark
a cellular memory, echoing and vibrating
and flinching the body.

Other people's memories are scraping
at nerve endings, getting across
synapses, revoking the myelin sheath.

They are dissolving the muscular tissue
that holds organs in place
and the insides are going sour with agitation.

In my grandmother's attic I find her purses,
small leather rectangles, tan or black, a woven white.
Inside each is the same thing: a lifesaver, a bobby pin,
a ticket stub from the symphony at Place des Arts,
peppermints.

In my mother's house the book shelves hold the books
and the books hold the bookmarks:
A History of the Jews holds boarding passes, recipes,
lists for holiday dinners, inside Siddhartha how much

chopped liver, how much egg. Buried in Thomas Mann
what she made, what was eaten. Howl has
where we sat, who came, what was put away, what the CBC played
that day. An archaeology. I don't take
what is flattened there. Just take it in.

Just This

A friend says she thinks we're not wired
for this much intimacy, for knowing so much
about so many lives. Last week I joined her
in the group she runs, all the women survivors
of violence: one-off randomness and deliberate
consistent relentless assault. She is gentle in the room
almost whispers and this is what she offers:
a space for them to speak or not, to cry or not,
to leave or not, to listen. It sounds cliché but the space
for pain is underrated.

A voice in me was crying: this is what I always wanted
my family to be, just this: a room and five people in it,
and enough quietness to hold all the shrieking
or all the fear or all the desire or all the love,
a room with people in it.

What Works

1. Index

Air. The art gallery and bank (of Montreal, Canada, Greece
on the Danforth, Korea on Bloor).

Bicycles (falling) and birds and beef and buses on Christie Street.

Carr (Emily): cedar tree, cedar pole.

Cemetery, Consolatrix Afflictorum (the stone virgin on a hill of sage in
Saskatchewan, all the stations below. Climb down to the parking lot, a
handful of fruit.)

Chocolate.

Cows and customs (if a cow falls on your land who is responsible?).

Deer (dead), electricity, gas, God, Ginsberg (to ease the pain of living).

Gown, hospital, hydro, Hyrtl Skull Collection. Food (another inventory:
duck, beef, deer, bread, white, milk, eggs).

Inspections, law, legislature (that building in the middle of a circle owned
by a tower), library (the subway under its tables).

Lunetti (Adoration of the Shepherds) and marriage (their bodies shine).

Military (epaulettes, suits, pinstripes), monastery (in a circle), news.

Neighbourhood nursing homes. Ontario. Paintings, parking tickets,
paramedics (Ken and Pete), poems.

Queen's Park, Queen Street Mental Health, radiation, red, Rothko.

Solid house (all our houses are imaginary).

South, subway, Sunnybrook shuttle bus, summons, synagogue, syringe.

Tattoo (a painting on skin or wall: eyeliner at the top of the CN Tower, blinking).

Teacher (Mrs. Martin, Ms. V. singing), tenor, tent (flapping, flapping, all my tent pegs banged in).

Trees (bloom), underground, voltage.

2. Demographics

men and women, teachers, hospital workers, politicians, people who
shop at Loblaws, cake bakers, people who are retired, vulnerable, lost,
who don't know the names of things, pretzel eaters, artists, people who've
been to any kind of gallery, who ride bicycles, subways, people who walk
on oily gravel roads, get parking tickets, pay, have fallen in love with
paramedics, people who are intimate with the mouths of flowers, people
compelled to watch the academy awards disgusted, who watch news on
television, people who want attention without saying so, whose bodies
fill with anxiety like a liquid, who love something that won't leave them,
and something that will, warriors who take vitamins, ambivalent people,
scared people who do things, anyone willing.

Work

How does it happen?
A person gives 43 years to a place
of work. To a job. 43 years.
How? It happens
one coffee at a time, one bagel
toasted. One pen at a time, one typewriter
then one computer. It happens one
mimeographed sheet of paper
at a time and one paper shredded. One
never-quite-up-to-par-actually-pretty-lousy
photocopier at a time. It happens one
more coffee at a time and one more
face at the desk. One story at a time,
one tear, many. One rage
at a time, one *thank you*. Somebody
else's arrival and somebody else's
retirement. Somebody's baby, somebody's
death. It happens and then
one more coffee, one more 2 o'clock
in the afternoon. One more lunch
eaten at the busy desk. One more year
of winter walks to work, one more
year of raw throats. One more meeting, yet
another meeting. It happens. Somehow.
A person spends 43 years of a life.
She gives and spends. Makes a life.
43 years. One at a time.

But then how do we say goodbye?
One meeting at a time,
counting down to the last.
The last lunch. The last time I say:
see you in the morning.
We count. Driving ourselves, each other
crazy with goodbyes, last times.
The minutes fill up with goodbyes.
We say goodbye with everything.
One story at a time. One tear at a time.
One at a time. One of us
at a time.

Goodbye to All the Rooms

She thanked the shower for its heat in winter,
its ferocious strength. Told her bedroom
she would miss it: first place she created,
indeterminate colour between peach
and pink. Burnt a picture of her old dead self
in the kitchen sink. Tore up all the rules and threw
some of that Tibetan dust off the balcony, thinking:
Where is home now that this isn't?
Whose arms?
Which pocket holds the fear?
I've been a person in a whole body
who lives mostly in the skin.
Before you can leave a place
you must say goodbye to all the rooms.
You must say hello to them.
I'm ready now.
This body with its curves. This mind
with its angles. These greedy arms.

Everybody's Birds

I am sitting with my sister
in the small orthodox synagogue
the women's section, behind
the men, her husband. A year today
their daughter buried.

Enter the substantial scroll wrapped
in a fine wine velvet mantle
on which their daughter's name is sewn in gold.
Her date of birth and five years later, death.

And at the front, the husband's
called to make the prayer
that brings the Torah home. Invited
to stand and hold the rounded book.

In his arms
the girl, his daughter, wrapped and sacred
cradled. He holds her there beside the ark.
The velvet coat against his cheek.

He is being held there too, upheld
by men in shawls, swaying in all directions.
Just as my sister, among the watching
women, sits alone.

♦

Nothing in her lap but hands
and only hers. She sits and
nothing tells her what to do.
The public work of grief is done;

the grief itself, unheld,
uncovenanted, alone.

♦

One year later: the paper-weighted belly.
Another breath inside her breath
pulls down, swelling
the gravity of so much risk.
And he comes out alive.
Grows up to be the one wild one,
grows up to be six
and chasing birds on the beach
till the lonely sand man bellows back
stop chasing away my birds
and the boy, in protest, yells
they're not your birds, they're everybody's birds.

And she, his frightened mother, turns back astounded
as though he'd yelled into the face of the stranger
into the empty ark, the ocean, into her face
it's not your grief, it's everybody's grief
and felt something lift, delirious, dispersing
back among the congregants, circulating,
carried
like the birds, everybody's birds.

A Possible Trust

A revised excerpt from the poem "Public Works"

A possible trust: if you exist
you don't have to hang on to it. You're just there
lightly in among the electricity and wiring and recycling,
neighbours with their lawns maintained
and yours patchy, in among the delivered newspapers
and the ones undelivered, raised to faces on subways.
You don't recognize words but there's the same photograph
of the missing girl.

You are there among the dollar stores changing hands
faster than dollars, and they exist too,
short dollar store lives, imagined fortunes mourned.
There too among the seen women with swollen lips, eyes sunk
at patio tables along the east Danforth which you never saw
before. (Do they see you? Can they?) What gets noticed
now that you exist too is only everything.

Before, the subcontracted sections of the world
were your provenance, you thought,
as though doled out in crumbs
by someone you couldn't see or could only see
like an emperor's photograph on a high wall.
Giving you to eat, birdlike:
be grateful but not responsible. Not charged but charged.
How the eye goes blank as the mind says, "Not this, not this."
Saying, "if I see, then what?"

That fear: to hold the small crumbs of grief
and not look up.

"At least I have this," the voice says.

That fear: to look up and be confused,
a small fizz in the head.

To be seen to be confused. And a madness,
a flood of answers comes suddenly, an avalanche

like snow. So now there is that small fizz
beneath a mountain and not one breath
for the confusion gift itself to fizzle.

That fear of revealing a mess.
Holding on to the tiny crumbs of poetry, private
conversations, sweet food, sadness:
these cannot be answered and taken away.

The loss of everything else.

That corner so small you backed into, that refusal
where you lived.

That fear: the threshold.

Water

One day I found a different life than I had before.
Whose life is this?
I had the dust between my finger and thumb.
I heard water rushing in the land-locked city.
I'd been hearing it for days, thinking
it was rain or a skateboard shushing
over pavement. Rolling on the land.
Whose life is this?
It could have been the roar of distant traffic. It was
none of these: neither rain nor skateboard nor cars.
It was water coming from far away, a fast river.
I listened as it got closer. It scared me.
I could not pretend I didn't hear it
bringing in its mouth, on its back,
in its wake something new, something like
terror when water rushes into places
it doesn't belong. Unchannelled, uncharted.
I could hear it under the high
sounds of the morning birds
the way you get warning of water
coming into the desert
and you get up and run because the valley turns to
flood instantly. But now there's no running.
A man's voice said the word 'shane.'
It sounded like a horse's name.
It meant 'pretty' in an ancient language.
The voice was calmer than the water,
and deeper. Whose life was this?
(Dust in her fingers, sand. The water coming,
neither friendly nor unfriendly, but
water, unmistakable.
And no getting out of the way.)
Whose life. On whose back.
What horse. What water.
It swelled and roared and cried and sang.
It reared and pitched
into the air.

Permiso

There's a tree in my heart
and I don't know its name.

It stands straight behind my breasts
like a closed tulip.

Permiso, it says.
Allow me.

The Leash

1. I remove my watch
   sneak peeks at the wrists of others.

2. Ride out to the city limits,
   plan where I'll get tired.

3. Oh, wild one, drinking
   coffee at 10 pm.

   You feel leashless—
   but even the word leashless has a leash in it.

4. How far might you go if you finally
   stop stopping?

5.

The Parade

Yesterday the parade came through
with the elephants and trucks and bulldozers,
the tears of stoics,
the train of dresses and naked torsos;
the twirling and the shy.
They came through here. You were there, you saw it.
You were awake, you even encouraged it!
And it came through, blowy and clear.
The horns were distinct and raised to mouths.
They were so ready to be heard, how could they not be?
And they *were* heard. No one missed them.
You invited it all through you during the day
and in the evening did it all again
with other people, all these strangers seeming
to know each other. You raised your arms
to a symphony, delighting and thanking,
and then—*what happened then?*—you went to bed tired, so tired
as though herds had run through you
but without evidence, except for the feeling
of earth kicked up or pounded down or both.

The Peace You Are Waiting For

will not come.   The sleep
you are wanting.   The space you are
longing to protect.

The body
you are trying to deplete and pump at the same time
will not do both.

There is nothing that will happen later.
There is no point saving it.

Time off isn't
about moments preserved.

It is not going to get quieter
until it is over
for good.

What are you going to do about it?   No one knows
what you are carrying nor will you get any points
for carrying it.

No one is waiting in the wings to ask
if they can hold you while you rest.

Grief Without Fantasy

What I lost
was not going to happen.

I had
what happened.

There was no more.

Preserves

Today I found an intact jar of plum jam at the back
of the cupboard, it opened with a satisfying suck
and plummy smell. I made that jam, had

lost track. Was probably saving it.
Stop saving everything! Julia Child cries
touching my cheek.

Poetry opens me and I'm grateful. Thank God
for Grace Paley. She writes with her heart
and peasant body. And Adrienne Rich with that brow.

Is it just the High Holidays or my age?
I feel both more
and less Jewish around them.

Spend everything! they say. Here, have a plum.
The old women of culture come back, feed us,
tell us where we came from.

Use These Poems

Use these poems as breaks in meetings that become tense
and threaten. Use them to alter
the wind in the room, the sail in the boat can fill
and go a different direction. Use them to stop the action
at customs, but be prepared to be detained
by Officer Deare. Resist calling him *dear*.
Use these poems as crutches for your eyes, splints
for the invisible bones.
Adrienne Rich says, Tonight no poetry will serve.
In the wider world, who has heard her voice.
Or fallen in love with a will that was understanding
and ferocious. Yoko Ono was not for everyone.
Use these poems to keep you warm any way you can. Burn them.
Their smoke won't smell of incense. But they will go up
and you will forget.
Memory isn't necessary.

It is late summer and the grief is in the field. If the husks
come off these poems and there's nothing there,
where will we go for food? All I really wanted
was to eat a little, rest, move my body,
love with and without fear, and lie down after work.
Hafiz says, Here's a pillow of words for comfort.
Take it, if it works, use these poems. Or leave them
on a plane, in someone else's bed, in an envelope
on the table, across the sentient grid.

The Spontaneous Poetry Booth

I went with whatever their whim or wish
what the look on their face dictated—
reddening with self-consciousness,
stoic and pale. Stayed
with whoever was standing
in front of me. Wrote the poem
they wanted for a dollar. Anyone
in my periphery could not come into focus.
I was stunned dumb by questions, as though
some other Ronna took care of that
and I was only the janitor
here to clean up
the stormed heart, sweep it out,
assemble the dusty detritus, the dog-
mice of the mind, and put them
on a page and hope
for a filament that would alight
in the mind of the person opposite,
the mind of the room
     as it seemed to become
               the poem
                      trailing out after them
like a gown

Molecular

I am wondering about molecular forgiveness
the grains of love that send us forth
to do the things we do. I am wondering
if that's in fact what sends me forth—
that level at the base that's also
the massive, magnified, overarching everything—
that what directs me is also where I'm pointing.

for the woman studying Molecular Genetics & English

Spontaneous Poetry Booth
University of Toronto, 2015

Don't Be Superficial, 'Cause We'll Soon Find Out

At one time, there was the death of a father.
At one time, there was the death of a brother,
and at one point there was a brain surgery,
and it was all just one moment.

I'm not just a feeling, I'm *seeing*.
I have sight and insight. And I'm
here committed to breathing
joy and painting, until there's nothing left.

I believe in peace with yourself.
And I need to hear my voice. I hear feelings
that are the truth of another.

I don't protest, I profess love
and the abundance of tomorrow
that I may never see.

for David George Thomas Shipley

Spontaneous Poetry Booth
at Brave: A Festival of Risk and Failure, Harbourfront, Toronto, 2018

Ars Poetica

I write poems for money
where the giving over
is immediate, before the fact
of the poem, before the hill-climb of heart,
the pillage of cells, the language
eruption. It is all and only
in response. The conversation
with silence tapped out
like an invisible ink, held to light.
The cash—a dollar or a hundred—
simply the glow I'm held to.
The person saying, "Do it for me.
Here is my door—will you
open it? Hold it
open for me to enter?
Will you leave me there alone?"
When the poem is written and I am gone,
it is in the hands of the lover,
as a lover leaves another behind
with the satisfaction and grief
of their own life, shared,
but taken back ultimately
into their skin. *It was always yours.*
I only held it up to the light, I only saw it flickering,
caught it like a moth in my hand
and gave it back.

Why Are You So Scared?

If I were chased from my house
by men with guns and sacks and flags
if I were bitten on the mouth by a dog
with a head the size of a typewriter
if I sat in a waiting room in emergency
with a gash on my hand
and a man came in with a machete,
if someone was standing at the foot of my bed
in the middle of the night,
if a flood swept through the house while I slept,
if I woke up to find my neighbours gone,
if the plane I was on began,
if the car ahead of me without,
if I was asked,

if I were in the street at night with a roar
behind me and a fire in front,
if I was herded off in a train
and there was no agency anywhere
to stop anything, not internally or externally,
if the crickets, firecrackers and flames
of sudden light and sound were indistinct,
you might not ask.

If my home and your home disappeared
and we were left in the air
with no protection from the air
then, with nothing left to protect
I might rest.

Appointment in Samarra

30 people in chemo today multiplied by
x hospitals in y countries and z universes.

Back here, H smiles through 4 syringes of chemicals, 2 bags of saline,
and a flush of life-giving killer liquid.

White-haired sisters in their 70s share clippings of their modelling days
with shirtless men in big cars, take selfies holding up their matching drips.

A woman in the corner looks exactly like what is happening to her.
Pale and bald like coal after a fire.

Slap me good and hard with mortality while I'm strong.
My body wants to run as though it's seen a ghost.

Ethel

I'm remembering that old game—
what three people, living or dead, would you invite for dinner?
I never answered.
I had no heroes. Or did not imagine
they would come. Today, Hafiz, for sure.
But the others keep changing:
Leonard Cohen
Adrienne Rich
Allen Ginsberg
and Ethel Merman!
I was looking for a politician or someone really sexy to round it out.
The closest I could get was Colette.
I thought: look at all those Jews in that list! A coincidence?
Thought of Beethoven and my old friend Sally Harman maybe.
Yes, I'd love to have Sally for dinner. I miss her.
She taught me to make jam and gin.
So that's it then: Hafiz, Leonard Cohen, and Sally.
If Sally can't come, Ethel.
She'd blow the lid off the place!

Rest

In my bed I'm restless.
I want a fellow moon to look at the moon with.

What is the old lady across doing up so late?
Hello, other moon.

Health

In April, Frank plucked tiny boatloads of sushi off the river
at the lunch counter, pronouncing "odd" the Thousand Island dressing.

This week, in hospital, he said his name was June or May.
Is full of tumours, clots, immanence.

"It's not that you're actually dying," my teacher said, "but in three months,
on the 7th, you're going to die. Put your affairs in order."

That night, a screen popped up on the computer, warning,
"This feature is unavailable"—and I misread *feature* as *future*.

Then Frank—healthy, robust, snide, scared, umbrella-wielding,
barrel-chested, heart-softening Frank—died.

He said, "Is this it then? Is this how it ends?"

I wanted him to live, but want has nothing to do with it.

While I was practicing letting go, he went.
Both made everything dayglow.

I noticed the root system in a plant germinating by the window,
watery waves of light, that little worm of growth, incandescent.

It takes everything to look in the face of all our vulnerable skin.

Another day, I read a piece of sticky tape on a wall: *Is sperm unlimited?*
I suddenly don't know the answer to any question.

In order to stall, I focus on clothes. *What is the dress code of this book?*

In the dying practice, I say, "What? No more me?"

I go outside tonight and look up at the stars.
When I see nine stars, I make myself the tenth.

Affairs to put in order...

Holy Moly, I had to be nice to so many assholes.

When I open my mouth in falseness, it's my hole talking.

I think of those men and me. Such sad children we were.

We wanted so badly to get our happiness from each other.
And failed.

There are things to say to each of you,
I don't know what.

Guilt is a reflex, but it's stingy. Try sorrow.

I will not have apologized enough.
I will not have fixed what is broken around me and inside me.
I will not have whispered into the ear of the world.
Unless you are the world.

What is a relationship?
Get there when you're with someone, and find out.

Flying hundreds of miles
over Midwest brown and beige, Midwest blue,
I begin to feel simply brown and beige and blue.

I am sharing the world with everything at once.

Fear rises—the desire for a hand between my breasts
to calm the flap.

This cusp has no *sp*. Only *cu*.

There is no *fix* for the *suf*.

The more dead I'm close to, the aliver I get.

In the past, I'd have wanted someone to lie on me,
their whole body covering mine, the way a blanket puts out a fire.

I wanted to be dampened.
Fire scares me, but dampness pisses me off.

I go out of my mind for a minute and wonder—*can I stay here?*

My body is a cymbal, not a symbol—there is clapping going on,
front and back, front and back.

I take turns running away and towards.
A kid who couldn't be held was wrapped in blankets.

A kid watched a train go by, as it vanished he shouted, "*More train!*"

"Tell my siblings I'm an angel," Frank said, "black-winged."

On the drugstore planet, everyone wants a spiritual six-pack.

Apothecary or *Apoethecary*?

Things I'd like more of: love, generosity, courage—*ya!*

Things to let go of: being chintzy, my bicycle,
the extra seconds ill-obtained, all the little filches,
clothes—especially the beautiful ones, any words with my mouth,
the two good legs and one good eye.

If I really loved someone,
the way Frank loved Connie, and Connie loves Frank,
would it be harder to let my person go?

Do I love anyone like that? Poetry?

Let sacrifice be my baby.

My stomach with its ignored, indulged demands—that's the end of it.

My heart with its frantic claims, my voice—that's the end of it.

Body of air and want, the only parachute is awareness.

Frank got quiet. I made poems.
Birds made sounds, acrobatic and peaceful.

There's a moment when you have nothing to say. It doesn't last.
Words can't help but come back.

They want so badly to be in our mouths.

More train!

Walking the Hospital

When I was seventeen, I got a case of hives that didn't go away. I went to the Montreal General Hospital. They did tests and asked questions but no one asked if anything had happened. A change of detergent, maybe? No, a suicide. I didn't think that was relevant, and no one else did. Three months later, sitting with a friend the same age drinking wine, she told me her friend was killed in a crash. And now we were talking. A week later the hives were gone. What I remember from my hospital visit was walking with the doctor. He walked fast in his long white coat and as I tried to keep up he became aware of his gait but didn't slow down. "Walking the hospital," he called it.

I see it now as a gait of ownership. The way the lawyers and police officers and criminals walked the halls of City Court that time I was a witness: like they owned the place. It's a performance of invulnerability that strikes me, when I see it, as awesome and alarming and impossible. Now when I bring poetry into the hospital, I say to myself, *Wake up, you're going into a hospital. There are sick people here,* I say, *pay attention.*

This is not the way I've walked into any other job, though I've been a psychotherapist at a university, and an addictions counselor in a home the residents called, "The Last House on the Block." I didn't give over to the severity of their needs, I was so anxious to "do it right," whatever it was. But now there is no right.

Poetry in the hospital has no template, no colleagues, no management. I'm always temporary, and I go alone. When I look at the patients and staff, visitors, families—the fragility—I see how I don't own anything, not my role, not my health, not my body.

The first week I started, things got blurry fast. I was photographed for the newspaper in a big *hoo-hah* of celebration and curiosity about a poet-in-residence. I got dressed in very unpoetic clothes, corporate, really. The publicity thrilled me with an identity. What does a Hospital Poet look like? I stood smiling in the hallway between Emergency and the synagogue. That night I was back in emergency in my sweat pants with my mother's kidney failure. *Am I the same person?* I stood around like every other nervous daughter. Grateful, terrified.

I wanted to give poems to the staff, instead doughnuts. It was then that I made that vow to pay attention every time I came in, to wake up and say, "Sick people here," meaning also "vulnerable people." The sand is shifting and the person in front of me might *walk the halls* one day differently than the next. I would never know who I was dealing with, or who I would be in response. Poetry was my currency, when I had access to any currency at all. Otherwise, it was the heart.

It got blurrier. Friends got ill; I wore Hazmat suits. Some got better; some died. There were staff who wanted poems for their patients and patients who wanted poems for their doctors. I prescribed poems on little pads. Some folks ignored me or politely recoiled. Emotion and poetry, two of the stickiest places you can lay your hands.

I met people once and then never again. I met the starving who didn't know they were starving, return customers in imaging, those waiting for results, for tests, for Wheel-Trans, for answers, for a baby. Addictions, grief. The repetitive patterns that embarrass us and ground us and return us to each other. Trauma, fear, irritation, compassion, racism. Flu shots, gun shots, chemo, ortho, maxillofacial. Coffee shop, gift shop, book shop. Construction, reconstruction, maternity, residency, redundancy, labour of all kinds. Kindness. Bed, toilet, tanks, chair. Wheels. Do not take for granted who will need or not need anything. My motto: Everyone who is alive could use a poem. Whether they want one is a different matter.

Once, in the middle of a day spent in waiting rooms, a friend texted that her friend had just received a diagnosis in the same hospital. *And now we were talking.* "Does she want a poem?" I asked hesitantly, thinking it ridiculous given the enormity. "Yes," she said. She did. I sat on the floor beside her. I'm not a pastoral care person, not religious really, but poetry forced me into something like that. I had started writing poems on the spot for people, a dollar a poem at their request. The conversation would drop from the realm of the social into a void out of which words sometimes came. In those moments, it was difficult to answer simple questions, like my name.

Wired into the crack the air made between us, I was plugged into something that didn't sleep. That's when I knew I needed whatever it is that poetry points to, the thing with feathers, the thing that *steadies* in the torrent, that allows the continued opening without falling in, or falling without landing. I call it meditation, but there are many forms. What do you plug into when you're suddenly plugged in and the things you think are normal have no bearing?

My mother got well, my friend Judy got sick then sicker then well, my back went out, staff went on leave, or died. The doctor who took care of the city during SARS was no more. The biggest wildest mayor in Toronto's history lay upstairs under anesthetic. These men too who owned the place, they were walking the halls differently or not walking them at all. We all walked them differently, depending on the day.

I wrote poems for administrators, the CEO, prescribed them for residents from Egypt, Illinois. Outside, the normal world got surreal in its perfect continuation. People married, held rites of passage. But the blur? What were we but action and exchange?

Early on I thought, "The hospital is my patient." But that's too grand. There are people having experiences here. Who you were when you came in is not the same. Whither either. You bring home a new person in a tiny carrier, or leave ones behind.

Then my colleague in meditation with a big strong chest died from the lungs. I watched. I wrote a poem. I was not a relative, a friend, not a poet-in-residence, not a health care worker. What was I?

He went down fast. His logic disappearing, his cheeks sinking into their bones. He was heading into a force that had no words but was palpable. Quiet and fierce. Like when people fall in love, the chemistry is not numerical. It was an intimacy. To be admitted to the precious moments of departure, to become aware that there is no admission, only a tear in the fantasy of separation, and a resting in what remains. We held him up until he flew.

No thing holds it all together. But awareness. Who is walking these halls now, who is writing these poems, who is reading them—and who cares? If each one poem, person, experience, identity, thought, bone, body—like a point of light—is just itself, does it need a story to connect it to the next one? Awareness, carry me.

The More

Do not let the day close down around an idea
of five o'clock, or a plan you didn't make that's
ringing in your ear. Don't let it close around a want,
a person, the shape an energy makes in your house,
an exhortation trumpeting the body
and making it run into traffic.
Do not let the frame of some picture you have
of the past, land around the neck of the future.
The future has no neck.
Just as at dusk, when I could not make out the paint
on the wall, my friend read aloud, "Time is on our side."
To which I responded, "Time does not give a shit about us."
Do not close down around the closing down.
It will happen in the anal crevices and the eyes, the heart does it
but doesn't stay closed unless it's dead.
Do not let this rhythm get on your nerves—let it
get *under* your nerves until your nails blanch
like leached grass, and a scream shatters
the closed jar of your throat by its operatic strike.
Do not listen anymore, turn the page.
Do not turn the page. There is no page.
No frame. No day. No closing down. No time on anyone's side. No side.
But the wounds feel, the screams yell, the grasses smell, the blood, the
glass,
the photograph. The frames are there for hanging things.
If you carry a frame, everything's a picture.
And outside the frame, more picture.
Outside the more, more.

Bukowski

One night my guy says I'm not mean enough
or funny enough to be a good poet. He's just read
Bukowski out loud. Bukowski can fight and confide
so why bother? I agree, but say nothing
which makes me no poet at all now, but a chronicler
who wants to sleep and is awoken by the wish
to be mean and funnier. To be somebody. Like Bukowski.

But when I look, there's a lot of flotsam jetsam
pains and wishes. My own shenanigans. But nobody here.
Nobody to be. The relief of that is like being let out of a jail
made of my own emojis and desperation.
Or taking my bra off at night.

"The difference between a bad poet and a good one is luck,"
Bukowski wrote. And having your finger in a light socket.
Bukowski knew he was nobody. That's what makes him so great.
Come to think of it, Emily Dickinson knew first and said so.
Everybody knows they're nobody.
Why is this such a problem for us?

Service

The doctors are writing poetry.
The poets are listening to the stories of soldiers.
The soldiers are changing the sheets of the aged.
The aged are dying as trumpetlessly as ever.

And if you could rub their feet,
that may be all you can do, but it is a lot.
Their feet get very cold where they are going
and then get very still.

Immeasurable

Today a woman of no measurable age stopped me
to ask where she could buy some meat, and her eyes
filled up with tears when it seemed too far or impossible
and every shop was closed. I could do nothing but stand there,
vibrating in the hesitant spring. We were just two more
meandering women going slow in the empty street. Some of us
looking down as though illness could pass through the eyes,
others looking up, sending out our million help me messages.
We stood there with nothing obvious passing between us but time.
Then she smiled and went away. And I thought of the four people
the Buddha met in his travels: sick person, old person,
dead person, happy person with nothing. And I felt like all of them.

Clothes

I took off my body like a shirt,
and what came out was also me, but empty,

for skin and clothes are just illusion keepers,
and maintenance is a lot of work.

So for a minute, I took off my corset-self
and went flagrant.

If you look with all your eyes,
you can see through to the garden behind me.

It helps, I find, to dress for god who, if present
is what everyone wears underneath.

Afterword

To Connect Is a Circular Thing

Yesterday I was walking down Bathurst Street, which is very busy and noisy—a steep hill, where I live, and lots of trucks were blasting up, everything loud. A bright hot morning sun and birds calling over, under, through the loudness—calling within it. I felt myself walking in my shorts, very small in all that, but there nonetheless, part of it, in it. That's how I'd like to write.

This is how I write: to feel (or hear) without understanding and to proceed. If I understood it, it would be over before it started. Let it be in process, let me be in the process of writing. Then we're talking about something active. And that's it too: a kind of talking.

When I was 13, I kept a diary. I wrote "Dear Diary." This phrase meant someone was listening. Years later, I read Toni Morrison, who says that writing is *deep talking*. I was talking as deeply as a 13-year-old could, and Diary was listening. "Dear Notebook," I'd say now.

I rarely have a specific Other in mind, an audience, a person, when writing poems. But writing from the feel, the phrase, the image, the word—and letting it go where it wants—that's what I'm after. Going for the ride, crying, I want to dig deep. And I find a lot of things funny. Humour is real. Even in darkness. A friend used to say, "Your poems show us what insides look like."

She was right for a long time. I wanted to take a felt-sense photo of my experience and say, "here, have this." I hoped readers might recognize their insides in my poems too. Some readers cringe at too much feeling—for me, for a long time, it was a release not to explain but point, to make a thing that expressed some version of me, and to connect. If there was recognition maybe there could be trust. The beginnings of trust. *Will you come?* I asked the woman on CBC when I was interviewed about writing poems in the hospital. So nakedly wanting to connect.

To connect is a circular thing. When I write a poem that works, you and I are in relation. My longest relationship is with writing. If there is no one else in my bed, there is a notebook or a manuscript. If I write a poem, and see it working for someone else—by that I mean it moves them, or makes their eyes start spinning—then we're talking.

This was maybe the beginning of writing poems for people (a more forgiving enterprise than you'd think.) People/we/I want first to be listened to, and that is at times enough—the diary listened! But to then make effort, intention, pull a poem out of the air and give it back is an articulation we can hold. Its energy ricochets.

Around the time I began to write the poems I privately called "service poems," my own poems changed. I started to write less about what my insides looked like because I realized they were mixed in with everything, and had no separation. More and more, I want to include more and more in the poem—be wider, the ache plus the streetcar, birds in the trees, and the smell of French fries. The poems I want are the ones that bust me out of the cage of self. They pop.

I want to write without my head involved. To go from play/fury, to write a word by itself even if I'm not sure what the word means, to include it, untrammelled—why should it not be here too? Find out later if it works to keep it. Call it passion or urgency. There is no idle poetry. "Have I given enough?" I wonder, when I'm really cooking. Have I been generous in this poem or held back and been stingy? *Will you come?*

As a photographer, I learned about composition. Once, looking out the window of a car, I said to a colleague, "Look at those trees!" He answered, "There's a problem with the wires." I realized he was framing his seeing, he wasn't seeing trees, he was cutting out wires. I want to see it all, even what I don't like. We have to, don't we? That's what the world is.

In Ireland, I began to exhibit my photographs. My first show was called "Mostly Trees" and it was. There I felt more relaxed. If there was an artist in me, I was far away enough from home for her to come forward. The writing, which I continued in private, began to squeak out. I did a series of photos with texts. The texts were not illustrative, but meant to offer a different angle of light so the two together made a third thing. I applied to the Slade School of Art with these photo-text works in my portfolio.

At the interview, I was intimidated by all these bigwig British artists. The principal of the Slade, Sir Lawrence Gowing, was sitting in on the interviews. He sat quietly in the corner while the others asked me questions. Then he said softly from the corner, "I don't know about the photographs, but you shouldn't stop writing. Because you're like a bird, with a very sharp beak and very clear eyes." The others asked how I felt when he said that and I said, "I'm shocked and I'm sweating." Humour to throw them off the trail. To throw myself off. Though I *was* shocked and sweating, it was a huge gift I had been given by Gowing: to have my writing read by a stranger, who was not there to look at writing, and to have him give it the most eloquent thumbs up.

When I came back to Canada, I had no darkroom. Writing was accessible, free. A notebook is cheap so I went that way. But that's just an excuse. I always wanted to go deeper into writing and was too scared. With photography in Ireland I had gotten too precious. Making sure there were no wires in the shots of trees. Now back in Canada, as I worked on my writing and began to publish, photography became the place I could loosen up. No one was watching.

In 2002, I went on retreat to St. Peter's Abbey in Saskatchewan. The last morning, a woman at breakfast said she was tired from waking up at 3 AM to write a poem. She was irritated. A young man, desperately serious, looked at her in disbelief. He said, "You're complaining about poems being sent to you in the night?" He repeated this incredulously as though she'd said she turned down a lottery win. That is what it's like, I guess, when a poem comes: like a lottery win. I have always felt that poems and workshops are a crapshoot—but not totally. There is a practice. I try not to wait for the gods of readiness to come down and drop poems on me, though I wish they would more often. I want to let it all in or out— associations, images, all my shenanigans. Plus, the harsh bits.

In my meditation practice, I'm learning not to edit experience. To experience the full fairground of disappointments and jewels in awareness as they swirl in. Once I said to my teacher, "I have feelings I'm not in support of." I try to write those too. I want to be raw and unfancy. Not compose, but see. To hear the words and not correct them. If red comes, let it be red. There is no better word now. Who knows what red has in store for me? Later maybe I'll edit.

When I think about how meditation influences my writing practice, I'd say it allows more of this kind of writing: writing wide open, including the pain and the soaring and a lot more listening and not knowing.

Meditation is not about trying to "settle down," but finding ways, practices, to develop stability in the movement. My teacher said, "You've been knocking on this door a long time." It was true.

Meditation evolved out of my poetry. And later meditation pushed the poetics further.

In 2009, I did my first Spontaneous Poetry Booth. Scared and excited, I sat myself in a chair in a room at an orientation fair at the University of Toronto with my sign that read, *The Poet Is In.* I invited people to sit down. Asked what they needed a poem for, listened, asked further and waited for a first line. Then I shut up and wrote. Tried not to judge the writing: not good or bad but listening for scraps of truth. I took in their faces, their phrases, the room and chaos, the things I could feel they hadn't said, and wrote. That inclusiveness was new. I wrote fast, they were waiting. I wrote fast to be faster than thinking that might trip me up. And when I paused, it was done. I had no clue what I'd written. A trance? That sounds a bit woo-woo. Entranced by an all-encompassing nowness with fewer filters.

When I'd read the poem I'd written to the person opposite me, their faces would often redden, they'd tear up or laugh. I would too. We were in *a thing*. What were we in? The only word that comes is awareness. We were in awareness.

It was like being stoned. Isn't that what the ecstatic poets like Rumi and Hafiz mean when they talk about getting drunk? Actually, I take three meanings of "drunk" in their poems: the literal drunk on wine, drunk on existence, and drunk on emotion. This last is one of the places where I lean and fall down a lot. I am an emotion hog. It's both where my early poems come from and also what gets me lost and overwhelmed.

The question I ask when I want to share a poem isn't "Is it too dark to share?" but "Does it still interest me now, months later?" and also "Would it work for someone who doesn't know me? If I were a stranger what would I get from this?" I am always relieved to have written even the darkest poem. I don't necessarily feel the same way if I come back a week later and go, "Blech, this is abysmal." I guess there is the therapeutic component and later the communication—the being in the world with other people component. The latter is the public conversation.

Compassion is not necessarily pretty. Its eyes are open. Those are the eyes I want to see through. And the poem needs to stand between us like a glass on a table anyone can pick up.

—*Ronna Bloom*

Notes and Acknowledgements

Cover painting: *Blue Grit* by Tim Deverell. Used by permission.

Thanks to McGill-Queen's University Press for permission to reprint poems from *Fear of the Ride* (Harbinger Poetry Series: Carleton University Press, 1996, 1999).

Thanks to Beth Follett for all permissions from Pedlar Press, and for supporting my work by publishing six books over 20 years. To Espresso Chapbooks for publishing *Who is your mercy contact?* To Tanis MacDonald for championing the idea for this selected until it became real. To Maureen Hynes for years of sharing poems and fussing their details together. To Chris Kay Fraser and Tracy Chevalier for helping me with the afterword. To Phil Hall: midwife, shepherd, editor, mensch. To my friends for your presence. To my teachers, Ruth and Jon for the practice. Thanks = Love.

To the colleagues, students, doctors, nurses, therapists, poets, friends, and teachers who helped me put together this collection by sharing your favourites: thank you for your enthusiasm and time. I'm sorry there wasn't room for everything!

"The City" was published in *Fear of the Ride* in 1996 and in 2018 was painted by PLANT Architects on King Street, 30 meters wide, as part of the King Street Pilot, a project in downtown Toronto to enhance public space, improve transit efficiency, and refocus the street to pedestrians.

"Here" is for Joe Kirkpatrick 1958–1980.

"The Job of An Apple" appears in *Viewpoints 11*, a grade 11 textbook published by Prentice Hall in 2001. It sits between poems by Robert Frost and Emily Dickinson.

"Personal Effects" and "Just This" were set in motion by conversations with Patti McGillicuddy. Extended thanks to Patti for helping me conjure the Poet in Community programme, and to Richard Chambers, Tanya Lewis, and Day Milman for bringing it into existence at the University of Toronto.

"Grief Without Fantasy" was made into a one-minute film in 2012 by Midi Onodera and was an official entry at the Toronto Urban Film Festival (TUFF). In 2018, it screened at the National Gallery of Canada as part of her Governor General's Award celebratory exhibition. Midi Onodera also made a film based on an excerpt from "Use These Poems."

The book *The More* was written while I was poet-in-residence at Sinai Health (2012–2019). Particular thanks to Allan Peterkin, Melissa Barton, and the staff, students, clinicians, patients, visitors, and family members who welcomed me.

"Appointment in Samarra" is in response to a morning spent prescribing poems in the chemotherapy unit at Princess Margaret Hospital in Toronto.

"Health" is for Frank Lawson 1955–2015.

A paragraph from "Walking the Hospital" appeared in a prose piece on *Lit Hub* in 2016 with the very heavy title, "On Prescribing Poems for the Sick, the Dying, the Grief Stricken: Ronna Bloom Explores the Power of Poetry in a Hospital Waiting Room."

"Bukowski" was published in *Literary Review of Canada* in April 2022.

"Service" appeared in the chapbook *Who is your mercy contact?* published by Espresso Chapbooks in 2022.

"Immeasurable" was published in *ARC Poetry Magazine* in Fall 2020.

Watch Ronna toss her manuscript here:
https://ronnabloom.com/news/2022/ronna-edits-her-manuscript

lps Books in the Laurier Poetry Series
Published by Wilfrid Laurier University Press

Kateri Akiwenzie-Damm
(Re)Generation: The Poetry of Kateri Akiwenzie-Damm, selected with an introduction by Dallas Hunt, with an afterword by Kateri Akiwenzie-Damm • 2021 • xx + 74 pp. • ISBN 978-1-77112-471-3

Lillian Allen
Make the World New: The Poetry of Lillian Allen, edited by Ronald Cummings, with an afterword by Lillian Allen • 2021 • xxii + 82 pp. • ISBN 978-1-77112-495-9

Nelson Ball
Certain Details: The Poetry of Nelson Ball, selected with an introduction by Stuart Ross, with an afterword by Nelson Ball • 2016 • xxiv + 86 pp. • ISBN 978-1-77112-246-7

derek beaulieu
Please, No More Poetry: The Poetry of derek beaulieu, edited by Kit Dobson, with an afterword by Lori Emerson • 2013 • xvi + 74 pp. • ISBN 978-1-55458-829-9

Ronna Bloom
A Possible Trust: The Poetry of Ronna Bloom, selected with an introduction by Phil Hall and an afterword by Ronna Bloom • 2023 • xxiv + 60 pp. • ISBN 978-1-77112-595-6

Dionne Brand
Fierce Departures: The Poetry of Dionne Brand, edited by Leslie C. Sanders, with an afterword by Dionne Brand • 2009 • xvi + 44 pp. • ISBN 978-1-55458-038-5

Di Brandt
Speaking of Power: The Poetry of Di Brandt, edited by Tanis MacDonald, with an afterword by Di Brandt • 2006 • xvi + 56 pp. • ISBN 978-0-88920-506-2

Nicole Brossard
Mobility of Light: The Poetry of Nicole Brossard, edited by Louise H. Forsyth, with an afterword by Nicole Brossard • 2009 • xxvi + 118 pp. • ISBN 978-1-55458-047-7

Alice Burdick
Deportment: The Poetry of Alice Burdick, edited by Alessandro Porco • 2018 • xxx + 64 pp. • ISBN 978-1-77112-380-8

Margaret Christakos
Space Between Her Lips: The Poetry of Margaret Christakos, edited by Gregory Betts, with an afterword by Margaret Christakos • 2017 • xxviii + 68 pp. • ISBN 978-1-77112-297-9

George Elliott Clarke
Blues and Bliss: The Poetry of George Elliott Clarke, edited by Jon Paul Fiorentino, with an afterword by George Elliott Clarke • 2008 • xviii + 72 pp. • ISBN 978-1-55458-060-6

Dennis Cooley
By Word of Mouth: The Poetry of Dennis Cooley, edited by Nicole Markotić, with an afterword by Dennis Cooley • 2007 • xxii + 62 pp. • ISBN 978-1-55458-007-1

Lorna Crozier — *Before the First Word: The Poetry of Lorna Crozier*, edited by Catherine Hunter, with an afterword by Lorna Crozier • 2005 • xviii + 62 pp. • ISBN 978-0-88920-489-8

Christopher Dewdney — *Children of the Outer Dark: The Poetry of Christopher Dewdney*, edited by Karl E. Jirgens, with an afterword by Christopher Dewdney • 2007 • xviii + 60 pp. • ISBN 978-0-88920-515-4

Don Domanski — *Earthly Pages: The Poetry of Don Domanski*, edited by Brian Bartlett, with an afterword by Don Domanski • 2007 • xvi + 62 pp. • ISBN 978-1-55458-008-8

Louis Dudek — *All These Roads: The Poetry of Louis Dudek*, edited by Karis Shearer, with an afterword by Frank Davey • 2008 • xx+ 70 pp. • ISBN 978-1-55458-039-2

Paul Dutton — *Sonosyntactics: Selected and New Poetry by Paul Dutton*, edited by Gary Barwin, with an afterword by Paul Dutton • 2015 • ISBN 978-1-77112-132-3

George Fetherling — *Plans Deranged by Time: The Poetry of George Fetherling*, edited by A.F. Moritz, with an afterword by George Fetherling • 2012 • xviii + 64 pp. • ISBN 978-1-55458-631-8

Sue Goyette — *A Different Species of Breathing: The Poetry of Sue Goyette*, selected with an introduction by Bart Vautour and an interview with Sue Goyette by Erin Wunker • 2023 • xxiv + 78 pp. • ISBN 978-1-77112-581-9

Phil Hall — *Guthrie Clothing: The Poetry of Phil Hall, a Selected Collage* edited by rob mclennan, with an afterword by Phil Hall • 2015 • xvi + 72 pp. • ISBN 978-1-77112-191-0

Robert Kroetsch — *Post-glacial: The Poetry of Robert Kroetsch*, selected with an introduction by David Eso and an afterword by Aritha van Herk • 2019 • xviii + 94 pp. • ISBN 978-1-77112-426-3

M. Travis Lane — *The Crisp Day Closing on My Hand: The Poetry of M. Travis Lane*, edited by Jeanette Lynes, with an afterword by M. Travis Lane • 2007 • xvi + 86 pp. • ISBN 978-1-55458-025-5

Tim Lilburn — *Desire Never Leaves: The Poetry of Tim Lilburn*, edited by Alison Calder, with an afterword by Tim Lilburn • 2007 • xiv + 50 pp. • ISBN 978-0-88920-514-7

Eli Mandel — *From Room to Room: The Poetry of Eli Mandel*, edited by Peter Webb, with an afterword by Andrew Stubbs • 2011 • xviii + 66 pp. • ISBN 978-1-55458-255-6

Daphne Marlatt — *Rivering: The Poetry of Daphne Marlatt*, edited by Susan Knutson, with an afterword by Daphne Marlatt • 2014 • xxiv + 72 pp. • ISBN 978-1-77112-038-8

Steve McCaffery · *Verse and Worse: Selected and New Poems of Steve McCaffery 1989–2009*, edited by Darren Wershler, with an afterword by Steve McCaffery · 2010 · xiv + 76 pp. · ISBN 978-1-55458-188-7

Don McKay · *Field Marks: The Poetry of Don McKay*, edited by Méira Cook, with an afterword by Don McKay · 2006 · xxvi + 60 pp. · ISBN 978-0-88920-494-2

Duncan Mercredi · *mahikan ka onot: The Poetry of Duncan Mercredi*, edited by Warren Cariou, with an afterword by Duncan Mercredi · 2020 · xx + 82 pp. · ISBN 978-1-77112-474-4

Nduka Otiono · *DisPlace: The Poetry of Nduka Otiono,* selected with an introduction by Peter Midgley and an interview with Nduka Otiono by Chris Dunton · 2021 · xxii + 112 pp. · ISBN 978-1-77112-538-3

Al Purdy · *The More Easily Kept Illusions: The Poetry of Al Purdy*, edited by Robert Budde, with an afterword by Russell Brown · 2006 · xvi + 80 pp. · ISBN 978-0-88920-490-4

Sina Queyras · *Barking & Biting: The Poetry of Sina Queyras*, selected with an introduction by Erin Wunker, with an afterword by Sina Queyras · 2016 · xviii + 70 pp. · ISBN 978-1-77112-216-0

F.R. Scott · *Leaving the Shade of the Middle Ground: The Poetry of F.R. Scott*, edited by Laura Moss, with an afterword by George Elliott Clarke · 2011 · xxiv + 72 pp. · ISBN 978-1-55458-367-6

Sky Dancer Louise Bernice Halfe · *Sôhkêyihta: The Poetry of Sky Dancer Louise Bernice Halfe*, edited by David Gaertner, with an afterword by Sky Dancer Louise Bernice Halfe · 2018 · xx + 96 pp. · ISBN 978-1-77112-349-5

Fred Wah · *The False Laws of Narrative: The Poetry of Fred Wah*, edited by Louis Cabri, with an afterword by Fred Wah · 2009 · xxiv + 78 pp. · ISBN 978-1-55458-046-0

Tom Wayman · *The Order in Which We Do Things: The Poetry of Tom Wayman*, edited by Owen Percy, with an afterword by Tom Wayman · 2014 · xx + 92 pp. · ISBN 978-1-55458-995-1

Rita Wong · *Current, Climate: The Poetry of Rita Wong*, edited by Nicholas Bradley, with an afterword by Rita Wong · 2021 · xxiv + 80 pp. · ISBN 978-1-77112-443-0

Rachel Zolf · *Social Poesis: The Poetry of Rachel Zolf*, selected with an introduction by Heather Milne and an afterword by Rachel Zolf · 2019 · xviii + 80 pp. · ISBN 978-1-77112-411-9

Jan Zwicky · *Chamber Music: The Poetry of Jan Zwicky*, edited by Darren Bifford and Warren Heiti, with a conversation with Jan Zwicky · 2014 · xx + 82 pp. · ISBN 978-1-77112-091-3